Own Your Massage

By Heather Leigh

Own Your Massage

Text © 2015 Heather Leigh

Before beginning body treatments, check with you doctor.

Everything in this book is meant to serve as a way to heal people. However, any information given is from a massage therapist and not a doctor.

Leigh, Heather, 1968-
Own Your Massage/ Heather Leigh

Also by Heather Leigh:

<u>Juvenile Fiction</u>

Hey Little Baby

Scout and Ellie, The Birthday Party

Scout and Ellie, The Beauty Pageant

Scout and Ellie, The Ski Resort

Scout and Ellie, The Giraffe Next Door

What Piper Peppertree Found

<u>Pre-teen Paranormal Trilogy</u>

Red Nectar

Black Licorice

Suicide Soda

<u>Non-Fiction</u>

Are You An Intelligent Massage Therapist?

Are You An Intelligent Mover?

<u>Blogs</u>

www.heatherleighauthor.blogspot.com

www.thechildrensstoryplace.blogspot.com

www.accessiblespirituality.blogspot.com

4

Table of Contents

For every client I have been blessed to work with.

Thank you

Own Your Massage

By Heather Leigh

The first time I had a massage I was worried and nervous. This was over twenty years ago, before it was accepted as a normal thing to do. Back then, it was either for rich men at a country club or people living on communes ready to read your aura and tell you how the planets were aligned on the day you were born. It was not recognized as the must-have, health-enriching therapy as it is today.

My massage was at the home of an acquaintance, surrounded by lavender, candles and music that floated through my veins. I was at peace before she even had me lying on the cozy, warm massage table.

When her hands ran through my scalp, I became an addict.

On becoming a single mother with two young sons, I wanted a career that would allow me to be with them after school, and to serve people. After one massage class, I was hooked. It became my way to help humanity, remain a sane parent, and have money for the great things in life: mortgage, food and chocolate.

Now that I am no longer a therapist, having moved into the writing field, I know that I can offer my decade of giving massages in publishing this book.

Love massage? Then love it even more with these easy steps to follow. Bring your body into even more enjoyment of this rocking world of healthful pleasure therapy.

New to this thing? Wondering what all the fuss is about? Put your seatbelt on and get ready to discover how good it can feel to be touched in a loving, caring, supportive environment.

GIANT notice: this book is about the legitimate side of massage therapy. If you want a book about the illegal kind, go elsewhere. This is about the legal, therapeutic kind — nothing else.

Let us begin the journey of a thousand massages.

Chapter One

What Massage Is All About

Ever been caressed like your entire body is a temple? Have someone touch you like your skin is manna from heaven? Delve into those muscles with the sole intention of relieving your aches, pain and worries? Receive all this with no strings attached, nothing but a bit of payment?

Then you have had an excellent massage.

Receiving bodywork is your time. And how much of that do we get on a daily basis? But the amazing thing is, this is not just a foo-foo pampering time. You are not wasting your money on some expensive toy you don't really need. There are no kids being used in child labor, no smog emissions screwing up the skies, and no animals killed or harmed. This is about you becoming healthier, and a therapist earning money — all in a caring environment.

Body Talk:

Before we get more into massage talk, let me explain what is happening on the massage table. When a therapist is kneading away at your tight spots and rolling down long muscle fibers:

Fascia is being softened

(pronounced fah-shuh)

By the end of this chapter, you may feel like you have fascia coming out of your ears. Please bear with me. When you know the facts about what is going on, you can understand why massage is so important to the health of your body. Also, with this great enlightenment, you can do things above and beyond massage to manage your own health. Woo hoo! That is worth my boring body health lecture.

What is fascia, you wisely ask? Picture an orange. Peel it and hold up an orange segment. A clear covering holds each of those segments, or wedges, together. Fascia is similar to the clear covering surrounding orange segments. The clear covering is NOT fascia, but acts the same way.

In your body, every muscle fiber, strand, and group has its own fascia covering it like a Paparazzi on Brad Pitt. Why am I telling you all this? Because this is the stuff that is really getting worked on in your massage session. Fascia is being softened like melting chocolate for strawberry dipping.

For the most part, the real goal in massage is to create healthy fascia. The healthy kind is strong but flexible. It allows free body movement. Water, blood and nutrients can flow through like a sailboat on the ocean with a light breeze and not another vessel to be seen.

To feel the difference between hard and healthy fascia, find a place on your body in which the muscles are tight. Most often, this is the side of the neck and the top of the shoulders. When you press into the muscle, does it feel hard? Then you are feeling hardened fascia, not muscle. The muscle is underneath the fascia.

Most people have healthy fascia in the biceps. This is because we move our biceps through out the day. Press into those biceps now. Does it move around with no pain? That is how fascia should feel through out your body.

Fascia is great because it keeps your muscles from falling apart. But dark, yucky things can happen when it is not being cared for. Such as stiffen, harden, and glue to other fascia on other muscles.

There are three main problems that spring up with naughty hardened fascia:

1. **Blocked water, blood and nutrients**

Think of hardened fascia as a brick wall. This mean old wall is blocking the nourishing liquids your body systems need. Massage therapists are coming around with kind, caring sledgehammers to smash the wall to putty. Once the fascia has been taught to chill, the liquids can flow with ease and pleasure.

2. **Using more than one muscle**

When muscles are overlapping, they can stick together. For example, while typing, using the cell phone, and driving a car, your arms are pretty much in the same place. There are three muscles at work here between your shoulder blades. As your body is trying to be kind, it will glue the three muscles together via fascia. Oh, you may think, isn't that handy. Now I can keep my arms in one place forever!

Don't get carried away in your enthusiasm. Because now, every time you want to move your arms, instead of using the one muscle that is required for the movement, you are using all three. Every time. Can we say muscle over-use here? Now you are all set up for injury because your muscles are tired from being over worked.

3. **Pain from nerves**

   Nerves travel through muscle and fascia. When that fascia is tight, the nerves going through the adjacent muscle are pinched away from the liquids they enjoy so much: blood, water and nutrients. Nerves have one great way to tell you they are in trouble: pain. Loosen fascia, let the floodgates open.

4. **Holding in toxins**

   Like a ceramic jar around the muscles, tight fascia holds in toxins. These are the toxins, such as lactic acid, that are building up through exercise and stress. You know the drill by now. Break apart fascia, let loose the hounds of toxins.

The list just goes on and on about the areas in your body that are being deprived of natural movement and health by tight fascia. Massage to the rescue!

Muscles

<u>Toxin build-ups:</u>

Muscles have their own issue to deal with, just not what we most often think of. Every time we use a muscle, it is contracting. Those contractions are building up toxins, such as lactic acids. That stuff can cause body aches and pains all over. The way to get rid of those aches is by flushing them out of your system with water, stretching, and, you guessed it— massage!

Massage helps to send those toxins on a one-way ride out of your muscles. The muscle manipulations are releasing the stuff you don't want. But you need to finish the story of horror. If you don't drink them out and flush them away, they can stay in your body. That is why you need to drink extra water after a massage.

A deep tissue massage that is not followed with water can hurt the next day. That and drinking alcohol. If your body has to deal with flushing out lactic acid, alcohol, caffeine, drugs, all those body stressors, it will go on over load. So help that temple body of yours out by being good for the rest of the day after your massage: drink your water and relax. Let your body adjust and feel yummy that day and next. You will thank it in the morning when you wake up feeling refreshed and healthy.

<u>Contracting</u>

The other naughty thing muscles can do is forget to turn off. This is called cramping. It is what is happening when a muscle is contracting and won't stop when you want it too. Just another two-year-old doing what it wants.

Generally, the best way to get rid of a cramp is by stretching the freaked out muscle. This sounds opposite from what you may feel inclined to do, but it usually works. A therapist can assist in stretching and soft movements to alleviate the pain.

Gentle massage, and sometimes even pounding on a cramped muscle can also help. Anything to turn off that contraction.

Sometimes, muscles cramps can be caused by an imbalance of potassium. This is common in pregnancy. I had nighttime calf cramping during both pregnancies. After I started eating a banana every day, and stretching and massaging my calf before bedtime, the night pain went away. If you suspect your potassium is out of whack, consult a doctor.

Now that you have endured my human anatomy lecture, you are ready to get to the good stuff. The event we have all been waiting for:

Getting the massage of your dreams.

Let the show begin.

Chapter Two

Who Massage Benefits

(This includes a section for sciatic pain sufferers)

We've long heard that massage can help us to relax. But then, so can watching the sunset or falling rain. And those are free, for goodness sake. So what makes massage so special?

Massage can put you into a deeper state of relaxation than even the most gorgeous nighttime sky. Why does that matter? Because most dis-ease is caused from stress. And in today's polluted, over-populated, tension filled world, stress reduction has become a requirement in the fight to remain healthy, human and kind.

Desk Jockeys

When you keep your body in one place, like sitting at a computer typing for hours a day like a certain writer I know, your body gets the message that staying in that position is what you want. So it will command the fascia to stiffen in to place.

Your body is not making this command to be mean and awful to you, it is doing what it believes will help you. That is the message, after all, you are giving it.

For example, many people suffer from **sciatica**; pain that starts in the gluteals and travels down the outside of the leg. Most of the time what is happening is this: There is a muscle in the rear end, about the size of pencil, that travels from the top of the femur to the sacrum. It's called the piriformis. When people sit on their butt a lot, like say, driving in traffic, the piriformis fascia hardens. On some people, the sciatic nerve goes right through the piriformis.

Oh, yikes. That means the nerve is getting clamped down on by tight fascia. And now we all know what happens when a nerve does not get what it wants: pain, pain and more pain. All the way down the path of that nerve. Ouch.

But here is the good news! A massage therapist can loosen up that mean old nasty fascia through deep tissue and leg movements.

Warning: not all therapists know about the sciatica/piriformis connection. If you are having sciatic pain, you may want to talk about what the therapist would do to relieve your sufferings before you make the appointment. If he starts talking about gluteal massage and deep tissue, you may have found an answer to your pain prayer.

Sciatic pain is a common pain, but that may not be your issue. However, the same idea holds true for many pains through out your body.

<u>Athletes</u>

Don't go around thinking that it is only the desk jockeys who get tight fascia. When working on a sports minded person, it was often easy for me to figure out their exercise of choice.

Bicyclist: lower back

Runner: side of leg

Basketball player: calves

Pilates: inner core muscle called psoas

Yoga: upper shoulders

The only exercise that never seemed to have any issues was swimming.

The athletic body will go on over-drive. Fascia will help you out by tightening into the shape you've asked for. Just think of fascia as the obsessive lover, ready to do your bidding twenty-four seven.

Stretching after exercise does two things:

1. releases those pain inducing toxins
2. gets fascia moving to reduce the risk of stiffening

The thing with most athletes is that stretching is treated like something to avoid like a rattlesnake taking in the sun. Stretching needs to be treated like sunlight, something essential for health.

When you stretch after exercise, hold the stretch for thirty seconds, **minimum**. Any less and the body goes into protective mode. It will hold the muscle in, wanting to be sure you are not going to overstretch it and damage anything. This is a trust issue between you and your brain. As with any trust issue, it takes time to let go.

Hold that stretch for the full thirty seconds and only then will the body say, "Hey, I don't think this guy is trying to hurt me. Guess I'll allow that fascia to loosen, and the muscle to be stretched out."

But lo and behold, stretching is probably not enough to prevent fascia aches and pains. This is where massage maintenance comes in. It can get to the areas of your body that are just about impossible to stretch on your own. Also, it works to minimize soft tissue adhesions. Think of massage and stretching like hot cocoa and marshmallows, caramel and chocolate, and pina coladas at a beach resort. Good separate but delicious together.

<u>Stressed, Strained or Sad</u>

Endorphins are the all-natural high. Your body pumps it out with no disgusting side effects. Not only do they show their lovely chemical selves after a good work out session, massage coaxes these guys out into the light of day.

So not only does a massage stab pain with a mighty sword, it also brings out that happy, go lucky feeling that we are often searching for in life.

This massage stuff just keeps getting better and better, doesn't it?

Even in you have serious fascia hardening, your time on the massage table will help you after the physical work is done. As most dis-eases are caused by stress, then having your endorphins released will lower the dis-ease in your body.

Feel good = less stress = lowered chance of dis-ease

No wonder we love this stuff so much. It helps the desk jockey, the athlete, the anxious, and everyone in-between. It's like wine and chocolate without a hangover or weight gain.

Chapter Three

Health Issues That Can Be Massaged Away

Here is a list of what the Mayo Clinic says massage can help:

1. Anxiety
2. Digestive disorders
3. Fibromyalgia
4. Headaches
5. Insomnia related to stress
6. Myofascial pain syndrome
7. Paresthesias and nerve pain
8. Soft tissue strains or injuries
9. Sports injuries
10. Temporomandibular joint pain

That's a great list, but what do those big, fancy words mean?

Anxiety

When I first began my massage career, I was stunned. A client would lie face down on the table for half an hour of rubbing and then turn over for the top of the body to receive its turn. Over and over again, I would not recognize the person.

Why? Was it because my brain had slipped into dementia without any warning? Or was it that the client had released all the anxiety, stress, and yucky stuff of every day life? I'm going with that.

We all play some kind of role in life: parent, spouse, employee, child, boss, crabby old guy in line at the grocery store. When you get a massage, roles slips away like dandelion fluff in the wind. You don't have to serve anyone, be a part of something, or put up with any crap. This is your time. With a 'poof', your anxiety can be gone.

Digestive disorders

Digestion occurs when we are relaxed. When you are at peace, your tummy, colon, that whole digestive track can center on getting its house in order. Your organs are freed up to do their job without interference.

When you are uptight, the focus of your body is on the negative. The body is putting out fires of stress, solving nail-biting worries, or figuring out how to not pull your hair out when faced with traffic.

Math equation:

$$\text{relaxing massage} = \text{easier digestion}$$

And remember: when your stomach makes what you perceive as embarrassing, grumbling noises, they are actually a compliment. It is then that the therapist knows that her work has put you at ease. What could be better than that?

Fibromyalgia

This is when the body has muscle pain that shifts, often has no particular cause, and can disrupt the healthy flow of life in a variety of yucky ways. I won't get into diagnosing or more description as that is up to a doctor. But what I can tell you is that massage often helps.

While it is true of every therapist, it is crucial that he:

- is aware that you have the condition
- is someone who listens to you
- has knowledge of what it is
- is someone you are comfortable with

When working with a fibromyalgia client, I knew to be aware that the pressure desired in one area was not the same through out the body. It could vary from heavy to soft, one inch a part. As I moved along a muscle, what felt good one moment could cause pain the next. Caution, care and vigilance was crucial to ensure a peaceful hour.

So in choosing a therapist, if you have fibromyalgia ask for a light massage to begin with. Once you have established trust and are happy with those fingers working on your muscles, then see if you are ready for a deeper massage. You being in a relaxed state is vital for a more successful massage experience.

Headaches

Now this is not a fact that I can reference, but I remember years ago reading that ninety percent of headaches were caused by not drinking enough water.

When I was a drunken sailor in Japan, a friend told me that hangover head pain came from the brain pulling away from the skull; there wasn't enough water in the head to keep the space between the two liquefied. I don't know if that is true or not, but it sure felt like my brain was sucking at my skull on such occasions.

What I am writing in this section is not from a doctor, or proven in research, it is what I found to be true after years of working with headache and migraine sufferers: they always had tight neck fascia. My massage teachers and fellow therapists also backed this up.

My hypothesis in conjunction with other therapists:

Problem

Tight neck fascia blocks the flow of water, blood and nutrients.

This puts your head in a state of dehydration.

This hurts.

Solution

Get a massage with major emphasis on the neck and shoulders.

Wow, that was easy.

And of course, we already know that massage relieves tension. So tension related headaches get the same solution.

I feel like Sherlock Holmes, solving the case of the mysterious headache!

Insomnia related to stress

So much research has linked the relaxation gained from massage to the murdering of insomnia; it feels redundant to even have this as a section. When you can learn to accept peace on a massage table, it is easier to fall into the trappings of a good night of slumber. There is research on serotonin release, sleep patterns, and the effects of a less achy body. So much research, in fact, that reading it all will also aid in putting you to sleep for the night.

Sweet dreams!

Myofascial pain syndrome

A therapist trained in myofascial release will gently release the fascia allowing your body to move once again without pain. This massage is concentrating on the top layer of fascia, closest to your skin. So the massage will be a slow, light process. The pressure is about the weight of nickel.

Does this sound crazy? A super-light massage that releases fascia? It can get even crazier when you are being rubbed in one area and feel the effects in another part of your body. That is because fascia connects to other fascia. Think of it like a knitted sweater. Pull one piece of yarn, and the whole sweater comes apart.

When you try out a myofascial release treatment, keep an open mind. The effects can be extreme, but will be performed at a subtle level. Kind of like flirting when you don't what anyone else to know you are flirting.

The relief you feel may be apparent immediately, or after you are done with the massage and tucked into bed for the night. If you have been extra uptight, it may take more than one session. Hang in there—results will be felt!

Paresthesias and nerve pain

Big words that mean tingling of the hands or feet. While there may be other causes that may need the attention of a doctor, it could be that tight fascia is once again the culprit.

I feel like the broken record therapist in repeating: the solution may be to open everything up through massage and let those puppies (blood, water and nutrients) flow like a flooded Nile River.

What I've experienced time and again, is that nerves are begging and pleading for attention. As they have no language other than pain to scream at you, that is their way to communicate. Like a cave man grunting out orders in a hunt, tingling and pain could be your body's way of saying, "hey, get down to the massage clinic and succumb to some muscle manipulation."

We all have our ways to communicate. The caveman language is what works for nerves.

Soft tissue strains or injuries

There needs to a distinction made here, folks, before we begin. A strained muscle has been overworked and can be helped through massage.

A pulled or torn muscle has been ripped off of a tendon or itself. If it is massaged, the muscle could be ripped even more. If there is any concern about which you have, strained, torn or ripped, consult a doctor before getting a massage.

Okay, got the scary stuff taken care of.

If your muscle was used like a horse carrying a load of cargo through a hot desert, it will probably hurt. And could have injuries. Gentle massage, and assisted stretching can help get you and that horse back in the desert of life sooner than if you just sit around and do nothing.

Often, too, is that the strained muscle could be hidden underneath a healthy muscle. A good example of this is the calve muscles of which you have two. I know you are aching to know what they are called: gastrocnemius and soleus. Part of the soleus is underneath the gastrocnemius. So when you hurt the soleus, it is hard to get to by yourself.

Massage therapist to the rescue!

Let her able fingers work their way into that calf and release soleus pain. Ahhh, now that feels better just thinking about it.

Sports injuries

This is already covered in Chapters Two and Five.

Temporomandibular joint pain

Also called TMJ, it is pain and tightness in the jaw.

While there are other causes that a doctor can diagnose, it is often the muscles that you use when chewing and talking (don't do both at once--that is just rude.). A therapist can rub the area just in front of your ear to relieve the pain and loosen the jaw.

If you want to go hardcore, a specialist in Rolfing or Structural Organization will get into your mouth and work out that TMJ. This is an intense, ten-week, deep tissue specialty to bring about perfect posture. Tight muscles in your mouth are released as part of the process. I was trained and have gone through this procedure. While it was a challenge, the long-term benefits were extreme. I highly recommend it.

There are even more things that massage can help with:

- Reduce post surgery adhesions and swelling
- Improve circulation
- Reduce scar tissue and stretch marks
- Lessen depression and anxiety
- Increase joint flexibility
- Improve skin condition
- Help athletes prepare and recover
- Enhance immunity by stimulating lymph flow

Massage is not just an opulent luxury to be enjoyed once a year on vacation. The health issues it can improve are astounding. So many dis-eases come from stress, and massage is all about relieving tension. By far the best part is that not only is it healthy, it feels good too.

It's like turning chocolate covered caramels into chewy vitamins.

Chapter Four
Where To Go and Who To See

The place you choose for your bodywork needs to be a perfect fit. This is a tailor-made, custom to order kind of thing. If you are not comfortable in any way with the place you have chosen, move on to what suits you better. This is your time, money, and energy at issue here! In order to relax, be relaxed in where you are.

Great news! There are ways to get a massage for every budget, atmosphere preferences, and body need. Let's start with the hurdle that often blocks people from making this a monthly requirement: the price.

Budget

In the luxury resort spas I worked at, the prices were huge for a fifty-minute treatment, plus a twenty percent added gratuity. Don't get scared by this! There are affordable options!

At the massage school by my house, the student massages are cheap, cheap, cheap. There are almost as many massage schools, as there are mochas at Starbucks.

Massage chain stores and local spas often offer great prices when you sign up for monthly massages. Not only do they have less environmental impact on your wallet, their system pushes you into following through with a monthly massage.

Many therapists working on their own offer their regular clients great deals to keep you coming back. Because here is the BIG secret:

they like what they are doing,

want you to stay in good health,

and care about you.

I know, weird, huh?

Another option is to find a therapist who will trade services. I used to trade haircuts, manicures, yoga classes or facials for an hour with my hands. While a massage is worth more than a haircut, it was a fair deal when traded for a cut for my boys and me. Talk with therapists you meet and tell them what you have to offer. See if you can negotiate something that works for both of you.

Mini-alert: be sure you like their massage before setting anything up! And, that they appreciate what you have to offer. Always good to have a two-way, happy relationship.

So whether you are on a budget or not, there are ways to get your body worked on without working on your wallet. A bit of investigating goes a long way toward better health.

<u>Alternative/Holistic Care Clinics</u>

There are places out there with practitioners doing crazy stuff, all in one building. The wildness can range from acupuncture, naturopaths and massage therapists, to ayurvedic energy healing, cranial sacral work and meditation groups. Let me tell you, this is a rambunctious bunch.

But don't be dissuaded by their non-western, far out there ways. There have been rumors of people being healed, feeling better, relaxing, and experiencing higher levels of health than ever dreamed of. Yeah, it can get outrageous like that.

Seriously, these are places that take care of body healing. There are generally different therapists with their own specialties each ready to help you. Kind of like a buffet of healers. You could sample each one and then decide which mode(s) work the best for your needs, body, personality, spirit and comfort. They are great in that there are options to choose from, all in one place. And the practitioners can recommend who might be able to assist you, if and when your health needs change.

<u>Day Spa</u>

Spa time for an hour or a day, mmm mmm mmm. What a yummy, healthy treat for body, mind and soul. This is probably the most common way for people to indulge in taking care of their body.

Local day spas are a great way to go. They generally have low turnover rate with their therapists because this is an awesome place to work. You can latch on to a favorite employee, or try out each therapist when you come in for services.

You have the knowledge that booking appointments are quick and easy, as the staff is available and ready to work. These businesses know how to take care of clients. Try out different ones to see which best suits your preferences.

The resort spas that I worked at were at the high end of the pricing game. But for good reason.

Included in your treatment could be steam rooms, relaxation lounges with fancy teas, cucumber water and fruit, Jacuzzi and pool access, comfy robes, locker rooms and exercise gyms.

The massage was part of your relaxation experience. Some people would even come in for an eyebrow waxing and then spend the rest of the day going from one comfort zone to the next.

There are also more services that are a hoot to try:

- vichy rooms
- mud treatments
- body wraps
- scrubs
- hydrotherapy
- Asian style massages
- facials
- manicures and pedicures

So when you fork out the extra money for the day spa, ask what other services are included. You may be amazed at what you are really getting for your money.

In-Home Massage

Tired of driving? Don't want to be seen anywhere near a massage clinic? Want to fall from a massage table to your couch?

Then consider an in-home massage. There are so many benefits to having the therapist come to you. After the deep peaceful trance you get lulled into, you don't have to wake up enough to drive. That state of mind can float you through the rest of your day.

Perhaps if you are a stay at home parent, you could pop in a video while the kids are there and snatch a treat for your self. Or if you work at home, it could be on your lunch break in your living room. Whatever your reason, having the therapist come to you is the perfect solution for many people.

Before the therapist comes, be ready. Move the furniture out of the way for a table that is roughly six and a half feet by three feet. Give as much space as possible for the therapist to move around.

If you have pets, get them out of the way. Cats are generally okay, but dogs can be a problem. When a dog sees his owner lying face down, he may think his master is being tortured. I'm not kidding! Even the most passive, sweetie-pie dog can get on the defensive and turn to growls, nips and even bites. So put the dog outside.

Think about your massage. Is there a scent that you want, special music you relax to, candle you want in the background? Bring it on. All of these things can be used later to bring back the memory of that great hour in your own home.

In bringing someone to your home, you need to do research before being open. The best way is through word of mouth. You will be naked under a sheet with valuables everywhere. I don't want to scare you from the in-home routine, but be aware. Know the therapist, or have references, or a recommendation made. It can be a wonderful experience but you want to be on the side of safety here.

There are so many choices nowadays on where to get a massage. You can get monthly maintenance that fits your budget. Decide to invest more integrative practices for all body health. And then splurge on the occasional trip to the luxury resort spa. There are just no excuses as to not giving the health your body needs to lead a better life.

Therapist

Getting a good therapist can be tricky. When clients complain about past therapists, the individual reasons vary. But here's the common theme:

They did not listen.

I have worked with some damn good therapists out there who gave the most awesome massages ever known to drift off the human hand. But, often, the massage given did not fit the request.

Here's a shocker: people tend to give us what they think will be good for us. I mean, it's part of our Golden Rule, right? The rule needs to be changed to 'Give Unto Others What They Want, NOT What You Think They Should Have'.

So when you tell your therapist to go light on the legs, give extra focus to the neck and avoid your pinky toes, expect that these things will happen. If there is a mistake made, like too light on ticklish feet, the therapist should change what they have been doing. If you say to go deeper in the pressure, feel her fingers prodding harder. This is your time and your massage.

Oh, but this is also a two-way street. If you don't tell your therapist what you want done differently, they don't read minds. Politely let them know that you are about to scream from their version of deep tissue. Or that the heavy metal music is not helping you relax.

Another big no-no that some therapists are guilty of is talking during the massage. You may have to tell him that you really need some quiet time and would appreciate silence. This should not have to be addressed, as we are taught the value of silence during sessions. Hopefully, a gentle reminder will be enough.

Try out different therapists at different locations until you discover the one you are most comfortable with. And, who gets the job done. You want to feel loved, appreciated, honored, and that your body got what it needed. This may take a few different therapists to find the one who is right for you.

One way to find a good therapist is the usual word of mouth. Ask friends, family, co-workers. Throw out the question on your Face book. There are more therapists out there than microbreweries nowadays.

If you can't find one, you must be living in a cave on a deserted island. Even there, you might run into a therapist. In the last few years, it seems like we've been producing them like rabbits on Ecstasy.

Looking for the best therapist for you is not a bad thing. I don't think I've ever experienced a massage that didn't benefit me in some crazy way or other. It is the best research you will ever do.

So, once you have kissed the toads of dismal therapists, and discover your match made in heaven, I advise you to stick with them. A long-term relationship can mean that someone is watching over your body in ways that you can't do for yourself. The therapist can see:

- changes in your posture

- weird stuff going on with your back
- tight muscles that you didn't realize were a problem because the issue just kind of crept up over time
- changes in your body that need further attention

Your therapist should be a match for you. The attention you will be getting from your time with her needs to focus on your body's overall health. In order to get this, you need to feel comfortable. The therapist needs to be licensed, knowledgeable, easy to talk with, and a clear communicator. Look around, you'll find the perfect one for you.

Once you've found your therapist, worked the cost into your budget, and are on a monthly routine, health and relaxation can just get better and better. I don't know of any other health project that feels so danged good, do you?

Chapter Five

Different Types of Massage

There are so many different types of massage that it is lovely, wonderful and awesome. It's like me in the cabernet section at a wine store — love that variety!

But if you don't know what they are, it can be tsunami-wave overwhelming to decide the best one for you. The most common types are:

- Swedish
- Deep Tissue
- Sports
- Pre-natal

Swedish You have probably experienced at least a Swedish massage. These are the ones that are all about relaxation, long body strokes, and gentle to moderate pressure.

There are many people out there who still think this is just an extravagance that does little good for the body. But here is what I have come to learn in my massage career: light strokes and soft kneading can

- loosen fascia
- calm you

- allow muscles to relax

- reduce dis-eases caused through stress.

In the beginning, I too thought if the therapist wasn't digging in to me like a sledge hammer on a tar road, there would be no benefit; that my money had been wasted. But after analyzing my body after light massages, and noting the effects on clients who like the softer touch, I was amazed at the health benefits.

The issue with pressure has more to do with what you are comfortable with. How are you going to allow your fascia to loosen? Does it take firm digging, or being completely relaxed in a gentle environment? Your analysis of the situation is more important than pressure level.

<u>Deep Tissue</u> — love it! The feel of those therapist fingers pressing in and delving out my fascia issues — mmm mmm good! Just lay me out like a slab of meat and pound me into a Pillsbury Dough Girl Softie.

In case you have yet to experience this one, the therapist pushes into your fascia, gradually getting it to relax and loosen up. The trick to avoiding pain is in the slow pace.

A fun craft to understand how deep tissue is working:

Mix a bit of water with cornstarch. Only a little water, just enough to make it like a firm pudding. When you press into it quickly, your finger will have a hard time getting in.

Push slowly, at the pace of the mixture, and it will open up to your finger. This is not only a fun trick, especially for kids, it demonstrates how fascia loosens. Slow and steady wins this race.

While many people are under the impression that deep tissue has to hurt to be effective, this is a pure, unadulterated lie. When pain is involved, muscles protect themselves and contract.

Let me tell you, it is not easy to relax a contracting muscle. We have to fight off the contraction and only then can we get your body to accept the massage. It is much better to go with the speed of the fascia then ramming against it.

Sports massage is done for professionals and amateurs alike. So many women crowded our spa in San Diego for the Breast Cancer Three Day Walk; it was like the Pope was visiting the neighborhood catholic church.

Sports massage is not just for specific events. Every athlete needs focus on his or her problem areas. And receive all-over treatments to keep in prime shape for their activities.

These massages involve assisted stretching, focusing on problem areas, rocking while pushing long muscles, and looking for ways to improve body movement.

If you are getting treatment before an event, moderate pressure is great. Don't over do the deep stuff because your body needs to be free of aches that can come from major toxin release.

If it is after a big event, the pressure needs to be light. As there are already toxins built up, this is the time to help your body calm down. Don't go on a toxin overload by adding more of the icky stuff released through deep tissue.

Stretching, relaxation and light pressure massage will go a long way in getting you back to feeling like going for another run.

Pre-natal, or pregnancy, massage is like having a play date with kittens and puppies. That uncomfortable body that may feel like it has been taken over by an alien force can finally experience complete relaxation.

Not only that, research has shown that women who had pregnancy massage often have easier deliveries and even healthier babies. Now how is that for a reason to become a regular for those nine months and beyond?

There are some crazy, far-out there rumors and old wives tales about prenatal massage. I don't even want to get into the weird stuff I have heard.

The most common rumor is to NOT massage the feet. UNTRUE pack of silliness. The feet are a great place to get the pressure you are longing for. All of that new extra weight bearing down can feel immense relief with some good rubbing.

The ankles are okay for rubbing also, but should be done softly. Many women have bloated ankles. Crazy thing is, the body is doing you a favor with those swollen things. Research has shown that the extra fluid can help smooth things along during labor. Don't ask me why, I am far from a scientist or doctor. Just be aware that feet can get moderate pressure, and ankles light.

You can expect to get a light to moderate massage. I know of therapists who think it is fine to give a deep tissue, but I don't recommend it. Again, deep tissue releases toxins and your body is already dealing with a newcomer. Be gentle with yourself.

Two cautionary tales:

1. Make sure that your therapist has been specifically trained in pre-natal. I have worked in too many places that put profit

over safety and let non-trained personnel work on mothers-to-be. Massage is safe but you still want someone who knows what they are doing for you and that precious cargo inside.

2. Do not lie flat on your back when in the second and third trimester. There is a major vein, venae cavae, between your back and the baby. The weight of the baby could block its blood flow. Being on your back is fine as long as you are propped up by a pillow wedge or stack of pillows.

Some therapists do the entire massage with the woman on her side. Others use a pregnancy pillow that you lie face down in. It has a whole in the middle for that expanding belly. Either way is fine. The way to lie is more about individual comfort.

The beauty of this massage is that you finally get to completely relax. Surrender your body to accept that this is your time. Your changing body posture, weight distribution, and possible months of discomfort need to feel supported and cared for. You need to relax here, woman!

Know that massage is safe for every stage of pregnancy. As with just about everything in pregnancy, ask your doctor before you do this, just to be sure.

The aforementioned massages are just the beginning! Add on to that:

- Thai: a series of body movements and stretches that a body worker conducts on your body.
- Shiatsu: stretches, movements, pressure points, and pressing custom-designed for your needs at that time.
- Reflexology: focused pressing into the feet, hands and/or ears that corresponds to different places on your body.
- Cranial sacral: small movements and presses into the scalp meant to realign the body to health.
- Rolfing or Structural Organization: intense ten week, deep tissue sessions to bring about perfect posture.
- Myofascial Release: light, slow strokes designed to release the top layer of your body's fascia.

- Warm Stone: using warm black river stones with massage to bring heat to fascia, as an aid in releasing tightness and toxins.

Those are the most common types of massage beyond the first examples at the beginning of the chapter. I recommend trying out Swedish first. That will give you a taste of what massage is all about. After that, feel free to experiment with the others. It's always fun to try new things.

Word of caution you probably already know. Asian massage parlors are often fronts for the illegal massage. Which is such a shame because true Asian massage is splendiferous. If you are in a regular day spa that is also offering Asian, they are most likely legit. There are Asian massage clinics that offer the real thing, just do some investigating before booking your appointment.

If you have more questions about the different massages, talk to a therapist who is trained in them.

Choosing the massage that works for you is a great search to be on. You can stick with what you know, dabble with a new one on vacation, or mix and match every other month. Variety in this venue is huge. And you get the benefits!

Chapter Six

How To Be Ready For Your Day Of Health

Booking

You know:

- Who you want to touch you: massage therapist
- What you want: a massage
- Where you are going: spa, clinic, in-home, etc
- Why: better health
- When: it's time to book right now!

Where do you look for your place of relaxation and peace? Internet, word of mouth, facilities you pass every day. Massage places are everywhere you turn.

Digital age, we are in it, take advantage. Check out websites of places where you may want to go. Use those search engines for nearby clinics or spas. Look for what types are offered, time length, specials, and prices. If a massage business does not have a website, then they are either crazy, or are still living in the dark ages of pre-computer societies.

Found the perfect place to try for a massage? Got your appointment calendar at the ready? Then whip out your phone and dial up that house of happiness.

When you talk with the appointment setter, let them know of major injuries, or a need for special services. You don't need to tell them minor aches and pains, or your pressure preference. Save that for the therapist.

If you are pregnant, this needs to be disclosed when you make the appointment. Don't wait until you get there to let them know. Some places require a doctor's note before they will touch a pregnant woman. And, they will need to be ready for the different massage that you will be receiving.

What the receptionist tells you about a service and what you will actually receive are usually a bit different. Most receptionists have not had all of the treatments offered, or experienced a massage from all of the therapists. They are often going off what they have heard, or even just read in the spa or clinic brochure.

If you need to cancel or reschedule your massage, do it right away! Most places charge you if you do not give a twenty-four hour notice. This sounds harsh, but you need to realize three things:

1. The spa has lost money if you don't show up. They could have booked with someone else if they had known you were not going to be there.

2. The spa generally has to pay the therapist even if you don't show. Most therapists are paid commission plus gratuity.

3. Another client could have taken your time slot and received their needed pampering time.

Now that I have given my strict lecture about rescheduling, I will be nicer.

Yey! You are ready to go. You've made your appointment, chosen your spa, and are good to go. But wait! Let's not jump in so fast.

Spas and therapists are generally sticklers about showing up on time. Don't wait until the last minute to google map directions.

I know I sound like a hyper-vigilant personal assistant, but if I had a dime for every massage that was cut short because the client was late, well, I'd be one rich lady. So many people think that massage appointment times are like making an appointment with a grocer at the checkout line. You can show up late, and still get the hour you paid for.

Nope, sorry, doesn't work that way. For the most part, your time starts at the time you booked. And, the appointment ends at the pre-scheduled time. This includes if you call a few minutes beforehand to say you are running late. There are usually appointments before and after you.

Plus, you should get there early. The reasons:

- there is often a health history page for you to fill out

- you may be sent to the locker room to get into a robe

- there may be a shower available to rinse off smelly feet and sweaty body

Getting to the appointment about fifteen minutes early is prime time. Take that as an opportunity to be relaxed before you have even begun. When you are already relaxed, it is easier for you and those muscles to accept what the therapist wants to give you—a really good massage.

Oh, and coffee? When I worked at a downtown spa in a busy location, clients would often rush in holding their double lattes. Your body does not have an on and off switch for relaxation. It is more like a slow downward hill on a path to peace. Layer by layer, strip away your anxieties and allow your mind to accept that massage as the highlight of your experience.

Take a few moments before your massage to do some connecting with your body. Any new aches, pains, discomforts? Sleeping nicely through the night? Are you in need of a comforting, easy going massage? Or are your muscles screaming out for deep tissue release?

Set your intention before meeting with your therapist as to what you want in your time of glory. I've had regular clients who came in for serious body issues. But when someone had her mother die the week before, another facing the prospect of having to lay off her workers as business was slow, and many people stressed out from in-laws visiting for Christmas, we would switch our time together to one of support, relaxation, and long body strokes.

Every massage should be based on your current needs. This is about what you need to feel healthy. So take the time before your appointment to reflect on what you want to get out of this massage.

Now this may sound silly and like I'm talking to you as a Kindergartener, but use the bathroom before the massage. Another way I could have been one rich lady through a dime collection? That would be receiving ten cents for every time someone had to pee during the massage. Just go before. The clock for your hour of time does not stop ticking while you go for a tinkle.

Leave the electronic gear in your locker, car or purse. There are few emergencies that can't wait one hour. The ringing of that damned cell phone has interrupted too many quiet, zoned out people. Not only could it bother the cell phone owner, there could be a massage going in the next room and that person wants peace and quiet.

Hopefully where you are getting your work done has a place to sit down before the massage and do your inner reflection work. If not, perhaps you could take a few minutes in your car before going in. This is the time to do some deep breathing.

Close your eyes, sit comfortably in your chair, feel the quiet space around you. Follow your breath as it comes inside of your body. Direct your mind to the flow of air. Feel it going out of your nostrils. Accept the relaxation and peace seep into your body. Know that your massage is going to meet your needs and exceed your expectations. This is your time for health, tranquility, and letting go.

Now you are ready to meet that therapist!

Chapter Seven
Talking With Your Therapist

As a therapist, I would try to make a connection with every client. Most people were friendly and also wanted to connect. This bridge between us helped me to feel what they wanted to get out of the massage, beyond what words could convey.

It is important to establish a trust. Even if this takes place in the time it takes to walk from a Relaxation Lounge to the massage table. You don't even have to talk. Simply smiling at the therapist and acknowledging that this is your time with her goes farther than you think. But most people like to talk on the walk. You might mention that you:

- have had a busy week
- have kids and need attention on you and not a screaming baby
- are under stress at work
- are on vacation and just want to relax
- are getting ready to compete in a bike race

These little tidbits of information can help your therapist evaluate the best massage for you.

Like, if you have just gotten off a plane, you will probably want focus on your lower back from sitting still for a long time. Having headaches? He will know to spend extra time on your neck. Running a marathon tomorrow? She may add some stretches to the routine.

One thing though, don't talk about personal stuff until you get to the room. You don't need strangers knowing your stuff.

Once in the massage room, there are some people who are totally okay with undressing right in front of the therapist. While therapists have seen plenty of naked bodies, it is uncomfortable to be standing around trying to talk with a stranger, as they get naked in front of you. Kind of makes us feel like a piece of furniture. Wait until we are out of the room.

As you have hopefully figured out what the focus and intention of your visit will be, you can get right into telling the therapist. When she asks about health issues that she needs to be aware of, you do not need to talk about the leg you broke twenty years ago. But if you broke it a month ago, then yes, let her know. Here is a list of must tells:

- recent injuries
- pregnancy
- rashes or skin conditions
- Fibromyalgia

- your exercise of choice
- areas that are causing pain
- what you want to get out of the massage
- if you are undergoing chemotherapy
- ticklish areas
- areas to focus on
- scent or essential oil allergies or dislikes
- bruises

Here is list of thing you probably don't need to mention:

- childhood injuries
- every pain or ache you have ever had in your life
- whether or not you are allergic to bees

It's not an exact science what to talk about. Try to stay focused on the fact that you have one hour together. You want your body care provider to have the essential information.

But going overboard in your discussion only takes away your time. The time with your therapist includes this evaluation session. Don't blow it with detailed descriptions of every one of your life's injuries.

But...

If you don't say that you need extra focus on a tight neck, the therapist may not discover this fact until the last few minutes of your time together. If you neglect to mention the eczema on your legs, the therapist might think it is something contagious and not touch your legs. Bruises need to be avoided. With dim lighting, skin stuff might not be seen.

If you don't want your scalp massaged, let the therapist know. Most people love this part, but not everyone. The biggest reason clients don't want their scalp worked on is the hair factor. If you are going back to work, a meeting, or a first date with the most wonderful person you've ever met, let the therapist know. They can put a light towel over your head so you can save your good hair day.

The number one question from first time clients is the underwear: to wear or not to wear. First and foremost, it is up to you. Most first timers choose to keep it on — you are probably out of your comfort zone right about now. No need to push to an even deeper level of awkwardness. Underwear choice is based on your comfort level.

The benefit of going completely nude is that your gluteal muscles can be worked on (aka your butt). Low back pain is generally coming from tight rear end muscles. That backside needs attention from the walking, sitting, standing, pretty much every thing we do once we are out of bed. If you are wearing underwear, it is a message to the therapist to not touch that area.

Don't worry about exposing your butt or private parts. The sheet will be draped to cover you appropriately. We are trained on how to place a sheet to avoid exposure.

Before the therapist leaves the room, make certain you are clear as to where to put your clothing or robe, and jewelry, and whether you should lie face up or down on the table.

Ready for your massage? Then hang on to your hat and get ready for the next chapter.

Chapter Eight

During The Massage

With the therapist gone, it is just you, dim light, soft music, and that wonderfully inviting massage table. Maybe even a hint of lavender in the air?

At this point, my body begins to melt before I've removed the first article of clothing. Just knowing what is coming drops me into a more relaxed state. As you float around the room, here is what you need to be doing:

- take off your necklaces and bracelets
- keep on wedding or expensive rings as they are too easy to leave behind or lose
- unless they are HUGE dangling things, keep your earrings on.
- if wearing a robe, put underwear in the robe pocket but nothing else. The therapist often drapes the robe across you at the end of the massage. Things could fall out, like expensive jewelry
- if wearing your own clothes, take them off and put them where you have been instructed
- get between the sheets and lie up or down, depending on what the therapist has told you.

- Cover your body with the top sheet.

Massages are almost always started with the client lying face down. When face down, your head will be in the face cradle. It looks like a big cushioned horseshoe. You'll be looking at the floor.

This is the time to let every single pound of you feel free in letting go.

The therapist should be back in within a few minutes. Take this time to close your eyes, and feel your peace coming out. Is there something that you need to feel more at ease? Is the music too loud? Want a blanket? Or are you ready to get those therapist fingers on your shoulders and let the work begin.

Every therapist is different in how they do a massage. The consistencies should be that they come in quietly and ask if you need anything before you begin. Often you will get a warm pack on your back, and a bolster for your ankles. This helps to prevent lower back pain from laying on a flat surface.

Wait until the oil has been applied and at least a few minutes have gone by before saying if you want pressure changes made. Most therapists will ask you anyway.

You want to talk as little as possible, as your focus needs to be on using this as your relax time. But that has to be balanced with being at a good pressure and comfort level for you.

The 'no pain, no gain' quote does not belong in the massage room. While there are therapists and clients out there who will disagree with me on this, I have found it to be true. If your body tenses up because I am pressing to the point of pain, then your muscles won't relax and let me in. They will fight me like a Japanese sumo wrestler.

And if you want a deeper massage, let the therapist know. Remember, this is your time.

Be aware that if you have paid for a gentle Swedish massage but decide that you want deeper work, you may have to pay extra. So be ready to accept a bit more added to the bill for the added pressure.

As you are lying on the table, feel like your body is very heavy. It should be sinking into that table. Let the therapist move your arms and legs where they need to go.

Let your breathing be normal. Be aware of the flow of it through your body. When the therapist comes to a place that has been painful, imagine the breath going to that area. Picture those muscles being manipulated comfortably in to a peaceful state.

Allow your thoughts to drift away. Two fun ways to do this:

1. Every time a thought comes up, tie it to a balloon and watch it drift away.

2. Imagine your brain has a volume knob. Turn it to zero. Imagine your heart has a volume knob, turn it to ten.

You do have some responsibilities during this hour of bliss. Let go of your stress, muscle aches and pains, and worries. The therapist can knead, press and push at a muscle, but until you let go, not much can be done. You are working with the therapist to loosen up that body. It is a give and take situation. Lay heavy on the table. You are that 'sack of potatoes'.

In Review:

- Drop your stress at the door.
- Allow the tensions of everyday life to come off like a peeling onion.
- Let the therapist move your body into place. Don't 'help' by holding your fingers out to be massaged.
- The only time you need to move is to turn over, and make adjustments so that you are the most comfortable.

Some clients will talk during a massage. I advise against it. This is your time to listen to your body, not your voice. Except if you are really enjoying this massage. Telling the therapist that you love it will only make them want to do better for you.

The most common sequence for massage is to start on your back. Major attention is usually given to the shoulder area, as this is where people carry their stress. Then they move on to your legs and possibly arms.

Usually, at just over the halfway mark, you will be asked to turn over. As you turn, you will be moving your body downward. Your head will now be on the table, not the face cradle. The ceiling is your view. Go back to closing your eyes.

You will probably get an eye pillow. These are great for not only blocking light, but also for relaxing your eyes. Day spas often put a warm rolled hand towel under your neck. Health and pampering should always go together.

Most therapists finish the massage with a minute or two on the face. Stay in your blissful state. Bring your awareness back to the room at a slow pace. Keep that peace as long as you can.

At the end of the massage, the therapist will probably thank you and leave the room. Take a good couple of deep breaths, and move yourself slowly off the table. Glide your way into your robe or clothing. Remember your jewelry and all of your belongings. Keep your peace as you leave the room.

Chapter Nine

After The Deed

The therapist will most likely be waiting for you outside the door. Be sure to gush over how good you feel (hopefully you got a wonderful massage!). We therapists always love to be appreciated.

Ask him when your next massage should be. If you have no major body concerns, one a month is the norm. That is a maintenance level. But if your neck is so tight you can barely turn, or your shoulders are up to your ears in stress, you may need a weekly treatment. At least until your body feels better.

The therapist may also be able to tell you where you need to stretch more. Or recommend ways to help yourself between massage dates. Finally, ask if you should get another Swedish, or if they recommend something else. Maybe your fascia could use the pressure of a deep tissue.

If it was your first massage, the therapist often avoids going firm in the pressure. This can 'shock' the body into feeling pain after the massage. But after this, you can dabble in the wonders of other treatments.

The best outcome at this point is to be able to relax before hitting the reality of your every day life. This is where the Relaxation Room is handy once again. If you are lucky enough to be in a place that has one, especially with some cucumber lemon water or warm tea, then use it. A few more moments won't matter in your busy life. But it will help to solidify your body and mind into this feeling.

Sink back into the chair and use this as your transition time. You just spent a lovely hour at a state of relaxation that is probably not your every day experience. Enjoy this. Linger. Let your body take in every last drop of relaxation time left on your visit. Having a slow transition time from massage to busy life will help you to keep the peace as you face the circus of real life.

Be sure to drink more water after the massage. Your therapist has just coaxed toxins out of your muscles. You need to drink extra water to be sure and flush out those toxins.

If you are at a day spa, take advantage of any sauna, Jacuzzi, steam room or hot shower that is offered. Hopefully, you have carved out time to do this. You paid the extra amount for these services, get in there and use them up.

When you are ready, check out of the spa or clinic.

It is a good idea to book your next massage before leaving. In our busy world, it is too easy to skip several months before remembering to take an hour for our selves. If the massage is on the books, you can keep up the health of your body on a regular basis. You won't face realizing months later that your body needs attention.

Also, in your busy life, you can have in the back of your mind the knowledge that in just a few weeks or days, you will be getting another massage. This thought can get you through a lot of stressful situations.

If you are at a spa or clinic, gratuity is generally paid at the front desk. Most places add the tip to your bill. Of course, if you didn't like the service, you can always let the front desk know that you don't wish to leave the tip.

Adding the tip to the bill sounds greedy at first. But as most people feel zoned out and 'high', the last thing they want is to worry about the percentage of a bill for gratuity payment. Also keep in mind that spas generally only pay the therapist a fraction of what the massage costs. The tip is thought of as part of their salary. I don't agree with that system of doing things, but for right now, that's the way the business works.

Get in a few minutes of chill time in your car before pulling away. Make sure that you are safe to drive. This sounds like my mom voice again, but I am serious. While I don't do drugs, after a good massage, I certainly feel drugged. Facing traffic and a freeway this relaxed can be like having one too many at the bar.

Also, keep in mind that the relaxed state you are now feeling can be had any time you want between massages. You can keep a mental feeling and picture in your mind of what it feels like to be this relaxed. The best way to get back there is to take some deep breaths and remember what it is to be at peace.

Chapter Ten

Between Visits

Now that you've had that massage, what do you do now? Massage can be a part of a new chapter in your life called, I Choose Health. Here are two options to keeping up with that new body frontier of feeling good all over.

First

The Peaceful Massage Feeling Can Continue!

After you leave that massage peace, you can bring back the zoned out feeling whenever you want. Here's how:

1. Take three deep breaths, long and slow.
2. Be aware of your body taking them in.
3. Follow them around like a midnight stalker.
4. Watch as they transform your body back to a calm creature.

Here is what may happen the first few times you try this: nothing. Then the second, you might get a moment of respite from a screaming baby or annoying co-worker. Each time you try this, you will get better at it. Practice makes perfect.

And of course, the more massages you receive, the easier it gets to stay peaceful. Because now you know what the peace feeling is all about. With each massage, the body bliss becomes ingrained into your system. It becomes your life reality — life really can be this good!

Use it as an in-your-face, get-out-of-my-life, force driven threat to anxiety. Thought massage was for wimps? Not many treatments are this hard core and feel good at the same time.

Second

As I have been harping on through out the book, massage breaks up that stiff fascia. Again, fascia hardens from staying in place for too long. And it can stick to other neighboring fascia.

While a good massage can help with loosening, an hour a month is not enough to compensate for a month of bad body stuff.

Some of the most common ways that we mistreat that beautiful fascia:

- bad posture
- repetitive movement
- sitting still
- exercise with out stretching
- funky walking

Bad Posture

Here's what we usually hear with bad posture:

"Stand up straight!"

That is good advice, but as Mary Poppins said it is a piecrust promise to ourselves: easily made and easily broken. Here is what I told my clients. Please note that this is not meant as religious propaganda, just an easy way to remember to stand tall:

"Lift your crown to heaven,

Open your heart to God."

When the crown of your head is being pulled upward, the rest of your body is forced into alignment. At least, as much as your current body state will allow.

Opening your heart to God means to bring your chest forward. This makes your shoulders naturally go down and back.

Picture a string tied to the top of your head being pulled upward by a helium balloon. Your body aligns to the closest it can get to the perfect posture you are meant to have. Doing this as much as possible throughout your day will add to the positive effects you are getting from your new addiction to massage.

Repetitive Movement

Repeated motion by the same set of muscles can bring toxins to that area, such as lactic acid. When that stuff piles up in your body, pain happens.

Massage helps to draw out the toxins, and then the body flushes them away. But you are probably not getting a daily massage. It would be nice, but then so would having weekly vacations — probably not going to happen anytime soon.

So instead, you can release those toxins through:

1. Epson salt baths

    Pour two cups of Epson salt into a warm bath. The salt naturally draws out body toxins. The salt costs around two dollars a carton at any pharmacy. You can make this even more enjoyable with a few drops lavender, wintergreen, eucalyptus or chamomile essential oil.

2. Stretching

    Stretching is like self-induced massage, pulling out hardened fascia and releasing toxins. For each stretch, be sure to hold it for thirty seconds. Watch a clock, this lasts longer than you think.

The 30-second rule is because the body holds your muscles tight when they are initially pulled as a protection plan against wayward, uninvited stretching. Waiting for the 30 seconds lets your mind know that it is safe to allow the stretch.

3. Exercise

   Movement breaks up that fascia. So move that body! Think of the hardened fascia as a sun baked clay surrounding your muscles. Rather than break the clay with a sledgehammer, you can do it through movement and exercise. Be sure to follow up with water and stretching.

4. Nutrition

   A good diet is easier for your body to deal with. If your liver has to process junk food AND body toxins it could be sent on overload.

Sitting Still

This is not about the monk sitting cross-legged in the forest. This is about the desk jockeys, commuters, and travelers, anyone who is hanging out in one position for long periods of time.

What you can do is so easy, but we just ignore the obvious — move! Find ways to remember to move: set a timer, do it at the end of each page or chapter you write, set up stretch times with a co-worker. Then at regular hourly intervals, do a bit of movement.

This can be as easy as:

- Roll your head around ten times in each direction
- Bring your shoulders up back and around ten times
- Use your chair to twist around and look behind you.
- Stretch out those arms and to that ten circle thing again.

Those are all things that can be done at the desk, with no one else noticing your crazy antics. If you have a friend or co-worker doing it with you, it will help with motivation and making it a fun thing to do.

So often, though, this is one of those things that people do for a total of three days. But if you think of the pain, poor posture and all kinds of gruesome stuff that comes with keeping your butt in one place for hours at time, well, the few minutes a day becomes a necessity. Make movement, even small ones, a part of your life.

If you are able to move with out being teased and gawked at by co-workers, here is a movement that is quick, painless and can freshen up some office boredom and blues.

Stand up, take a full deep breath, and drop dramatically from the waist. Feel like a marionette whose master has just released the upper body strings. With your head now facing your knees, and arms hanging to the floor, take three more long breaths. Your body will sink in to this and feel lovely. Then, roll up slowly, vertebrae by vertebrae, arms still hanging.

CAUTION: Doing this three times through out the day will cause the body to go into refresh feel good mode. You have been warned.

Exercise Without Stretching

This is like bicycling through busy streets without a helmet. I've seen people do it and wondered how long until they show up at the hospital emergency room. And don't call me a wuss. How many of you have bungee jumped off a hot air balloon?

While it is always better (with doctor's consent, of course) to embark in cardio activities or weight exercises than nothing at all, you need to end your sessions with stretching.

During your activities, your muscles build up toxins like lactic acid. Stretching and water helps to get those toxins out like cattle being called in for suppertime. Unless you have a paid massage therapist following you around, stretch out those muscles at the end of every work out.

<u>Funky Walking</u>

You may have perfect posture but then walk with your feet turned out or knees bowed. And once again, your body will try to help you. It will stiffen the appropriate fascia to make it easier for you to continue in your lawless ways.

Plus, you will most likely be twisting and pulling ligaments and tendons. Those guys are not supposed to stretched. They are there to keep your muscles and bones attached. You want your bones to be kept in place, not dangling around like a ball of yarn with a kitten.

Here's a trick to see if you are walking at least closely to the correct way your body is supposed to be. It is not fool proof, only an indication.

Start walking. Look down at your feet. Are your toes pointing forward? Usually, they are not. Most often they are going out or inwards.

In or out, you are twisting ankle, knee and hips in a way that is not kosher with a completely healthy body. You are putting stress on joints that are supposed to be living in a peaceful environment.

Try walking with your feet pointed straightforward. Does this feel funny? It's how you should be walking.

I fixed my funky walk with shoe inserts fitted by a professional orthopedics guy. The kinds you buy in regular stores are a one size fits all that don't really fit everybody. They can do good, or harm. Not worth the risk.

After getting my inserts, I started watching how I walked. Yes, I looked like a geek, watching my toes and ignoring the road ahead, but eventually it worked. Now I walk straight ahead and my knees feel so much better.

By the way, do I really have to add that when you walk staring down at your feet, be sure that you are not in an area where you could trip on a cat, fall down a storm drain, or fall down a thousand foot waterfall? Please be careful with your foot-gazed walk.

My way of getting out of the funky walk is just one suggestion. Ask a doctor, physical therapist or chiropractor if you think this is an issue for you.

So we've rambled on and on about what to do between treatments. You may be asking your self, well, who the heck cares about the in-between massage times? Well, I guess because it's like this: life is meant to be enjoyed.

Didn't anyone tell you that living in a body that is as healthy as can be at this time, is a good thing? You can get more out of the years spent on earth when you can move with the groovy tunes of what life has to offer. And always keep in mind that the next massage is less than a month away!

Chapter Eleven
What We Really Want From a Massage

We want to feel like our body is wanted. That another person finds it beautiful. That no matter how much fat has accumulated, pimples are present, dry skin flakes you are covered in, and wrinkles abound, our body is lovable. And not just loved for sex, but a truly magnificent work of art — sculptured by the greatest artist. We want to be touched, revered, and loved for who we are.

Yes, massage is relaxing, healthy, and can ease aches, pains, and dis-ease. But it is so much more than that. It is about you being cared for in a supportive, trusting, caring environment.

Each time I would walk into a room with a person lying face down, naked under a sheet, vulnerable to a therapist they had only known for a few minutes, I would be so thankful for their trust in me. This was a person who was willing to allow me to touch them, heal them, send them love, health and support. What a gift they were giving me!

The other therapists I worked with would often come in with their own stresses. But they would be excited to serve a client in need. The therapist would have an hour to forget their troubles. They would feel their own problems slipping away like melting chocolate. Backwards as it may seem on the surface, to serve another human being through a therapeutic massage can be better than an hour frolicking in a cool stream on an ultra hot day.

So when you climb on that massage table, fold into clean sheets, and lay your body to rest, you are helping everyone in that room.

Now let's be honest about sex. Yes, it feels wonderful. If it doesn't, then that is an issue you seriously need to investigate. But for many couples, the entire body is not covered in the act. Just the essentials are looked after, even in foreplay. The limbs, toes, elbows and ears are ignored.

And forget about a scalp massage. Ever had a lover lightly press your temples, massage each finger, rub all around your shoulder blade? Massage is your chance to get that and more, by someone trained to do it just to your liking.

Now that you know how to own your massage, go get one. I wish you the best of healthy massages with a lifetime of more to come!

Namaste,

The light in me recognizes the light within you.